Esophagectomy Post Surgical Guide: Questions and Answers

Esophageal Cancer Education Foundation

authorHOUSE®

AuthorHouse™
1663 Liberty Drive
Bloomington, IN 47403
www.authorhouse.com
Phone: 1-800-839-8640

First published by AuthorHouse   11/29/2011

ISBN: 978-1-4685-0531-3 (sc)
ISBN: 978-1-4685-0530-6 (ebk)

Library of Congress Control Number: 2011961027

Printed in the United States of America

Any people depicted in stock imagery provided by Thinkstock are models, and such images are being used for illustrative purposes only.
Certain stock imagery © Thinkstock.

This book is printed on acid-free paper.

Dedication

This guide is dedicated to the patients who we have encountered as we continue our journey through this disease. Our hope and dream is to give patients who are recovering from this surgery a guide that will make that journey easier to understand, less stressful and to improve their overall quality of life.

Contents

19. Does posture and the clothes I wear impact my digestive system?
20. How many meals a day should I eat?
21. How much liquid should I take with each meal?
22. How much liquid should I consume each day?
23. How will milk products affect me?
24. What foods can I eat?
25. Should I maintain a food diary?
26. I hear so much about green tea. Should I use it?
27. How much time should I abstain from eating before I go to bed?
28. Are there any foods that I should stay away from before I go to bed?
29. Will I ever be able to eat my normal three meals a day and be able to maintain my weight or even gain weight?
30. Should I take Supplements?
31. Will I be able to go out to dinner and enjoy a meal?
32. Can I take glass of wine with dinner?
33. Did I receive sample menus or nutrition information that will help in my recovery?
34. What liquids should I stay away from?
35. I find my food going down my esophagus slowly. Should this be a concern?
36. What is dilation?
37. I feel bloated after I eat. Is there something I can do to avoid this feeling?
38. What is dumping syndrome?
39. What do I do when a dumping episode occurs?

40. Why do I need to sleep on an angle?
41. What are the ways that I can achieve this 30 to 40 degree angle while I sleep?
42. Where can I get an adjustable bed?
43. Does my health insurance cover my adjustable bed costs?
44. What do I do when I travel? How will I achieve this desired 30-40 degree level?
45. Where can I get an inflatable wedge?
46. Does my health insurance cover my inflatable wedge cost?

47. Can I sleep on my side?
48. Can I sleep on my stomach?
49. I am tired after I eat a meal. Should I lay-down and rest?

50. Can I become depressed when I return home from the hospital?
51. What are symptoms of depression?
52. What Treatments are available for depression?
53. How can I stay positive during my recovery?
55. I am having problems with sexual interest and activity. What should I do?
56. I continue to think about a recurrence. Is that Normal? How do I handle the possibility of recurrence?
57. I feel a lack of interest in taking charge of my journey through the recovery process. Should I be concerned?
58. Will I ever feel normal again?
59. How should I approach life once I am home from the hospital?
60. What role does my spiritual side play in my recovery process?
61. What role should my family play in my recovery process?
62. Does my positive or negative thinking impact my recovery?
63. What is the course of action once a recurrence is determined?
64. How many difference chemo drugs are available to the Oncologist in determining the plan for a specific patient?
65. Are there research projects that are close that will be a breakthrough with esophageal cancer recurrences?
66. Have certain drugs shown promise in this area?
67. Are there other countries outside of the United States that are addressing prevention of recurrence projects?
68. I find it hard to concentrate. How do I correct this?
69. I can't seem to read and retain what I am reading. Is this normal?

70. What will happen if I pick up something heavy?
71. I have nausea. Is there a medicine I can take?
72. I have a shortness of breath when I bend over? Is there something I can do to eliminate this shortness of breath?

Forward

The purpose of this guide is to provide information concerning issues that may confront a patient during their recovery from esophagectomy surgery. It is intended to be a quality of life document and a starting point for patients and caregivers so they may better understand what the patient is experiencing. The patient and caregiver can use this information in discussions with the patient's doctor to help determine a course of action that can be taken to handle the issue under consideration. A patient or caregiver should not act on any information contained in this document without first speaking to his or her doctor.

Acknowledgements

We want to thank Bart Frazzitta, President of the Esophageal Cancer Education Foundation (ECEF) for sharing his experiences as a patient who has been through chemotherapy, radiation therapy and esophagectomy surgery in the year 2000. Since his surgery Bart has spoken to many patients who have been diagnosed and treated for esophageal cancer and he has drawn on those discussions and his own experience in preparing this guide.

Bart was a co-author of the book 100 Questions & Answers about Esophageal Cancer and it is his belief that this guide will cover the remaining information that all esophageal cancer patients and caregivers should have available to them as their journey continues through the recovery process.

In addition, we want to thank the Medical Advisory Committee of ECEF and members of their staff with special acknowledgement to:

      Dr. Manjit Bains—Surgeon
      Dr. David Tom Cooke—Surgeon
      Dr. Raja Flores—Surgeon
      Dr. Hans Gerdes—Gastroenterologist
      Dr. David Ilson—Medical Oncologist
      Dr. Bernard Park—Surgeon
      Dr. Martin Karpeh—Surgeon
      Jessica Harvey-Taylor—PA-C

We also want to acknowledge Ms. Letitia Sandrock—Psy.D as she was the leading force in dealing with most of the questions and answers in the Emotional Issues Chapter of this guide.

Last but certainly not least, we want to thank the Verdi family (Peggy, Rich, Zachary) and John "Popper" Keane (EC patient) for their help in putting this guide together and assisting in the formation and editing process.

FIRST FEW MONTHS POST SURGERY

"GOING HOME"

"Having a positive attitude about life in general will help in your recovery process"

In this first chapter we capture those issues that will cover all aspects of your recovery process be it Nutrition, Sleep, Exercise, Emotional and Physical Issues that you may experience in the first few months of recovery. The first few months are extremely important so as to get on the right path and move positively through this portion of your recovery effort.

You should leave the hospital with any medications that your doctor has prescribed. You will either have the actual medication or a prescription that should be filled immediately. If you entered the hospital taking medication for a pre-existing condition, make sure your doctor is aware of that and ask if you should continue taking that medication. For new medications prescribed as a result of your therapy and surgery, be sure to ask any questions necessary so that you are fully clear on what each medication is, what it's for and how to properly take it.

If you are leaving the hospital with an open wound, make sure that a visiting nurse service has been prescribed and scheduled to begin monitoring that wound.

Your surgeon will want to see you within a short period of time to ensure you are recovering properly and without complications. Your surgeon will outline their course of action and time frame for releasing you to your regular doctor or medical oncologist. If you are unclear about this plan, ask whatever questions are necessary to make the process clear in your mind.

For many patients the news that they are being discharged leaves them with a feeling that their long ordeal is over, and that they can begin to relax. The reality, however, is somewhat different and in many respects you are merely beginning another leg in your journey to recovery. At this point it is tremendously important to focus on recovery and remain positive and motivated as you enter this stage. Your goal should be to recover to 70% of your pre-surgical physical condition within the first 2-3 months after returning home. Unless you have complications this is a realistic time frame to use as a goal.

Eating, sleeping, exercising, overall physical and emotional issues will all play a role in your recovery process. Recognizing each unique circumstance and being able to understand it and find how to deal with it effectively will become a part of your daily routine. Certain changes in your body may carry the description as being a, "different normal" and you can either learn why those changes occurred and how to manage them or you can continually fight them which will be frustrating and counter-productive.

Each of the areas mentioned above will play a role in your total recovery and it is critically important that you focus on each area to the extent that you minimize the related issue and its impact on your life to the greatest extent possible.

The routine of walking, breathing and coughing exercises that you began in the hospital must continue at home if you intend to recover quickly. What you will find is that you must be more self-motivating as you will no longer have a nurse reminding you to walk, reminding you to use the breathing machine or to do your coughing exercises.

We found that exercising had a profound impact on your recovery process and on your emotional state. At one point, you may come to the realization that you have become a "Couch Potato". If you don't want to exercise and often used the excuse that you are tired now and if you were to exercise you would be even more tired and so, you would do nothing. This vicious cycle is completely counter productive for a post surgical patient in that exercising has a way of improving various aspects of your recovery process. Exercise will improve your appetite, speed healing of your surgical sites and lessen pain. It will also improve your lung capacity and your overall feeling of being in good health.

At this point it is critical to carefully monitor your weight. Your weight must be stabilized and over the first six months after discharge you should begin slowly regaining some of the weight lost during therapy and surgery. In some cases patients who were overweight prior to diagnosis may not want to gain all of their weight back. It is important to consult with a nutritionist to determine a proper goal weight and work towards that objective. What is important during this period is that the patient, not continue to lose weight. Any continuous weight loss requires medical intervention to determine its cause and a plan of action to reverse losing weight should be implemented.

Exercising Issues

One of the more critical activities you should definitely plan to do is exercise. During the first few months of recovery exercising will help in various ways. It will help you heal sooner, you will get your appetite back quicker and exercising will have a positive impact on your mind and your ability to recover in a shorter period of time.

You should consult your doctor as to the exercise plan you should implement. On average walking 1 ½ miles, 3 times a week at a pace that will give you a cardio vascular type workout should suffice.

Please check the chapter on physical issues contained in this guide for further information on this topic.

Nutritional Issues

Eating will be a challenge for you when you leave the hospital. Because more than likely they took a part of your stomach away when they did the surgery you will have a smaller stomach but yet you will need the same amount of calories you took in when you were with a full stomach before the surgery. The Institution that you were treated at may send a menu plan for you to use for a given amount of time as you begin your recovery process. The transition from fluids, to a soft mechanical to a full menu of foods should be adhered to as it will play a major role in your eating ability as you go further out in your recovery process.

In order to get the amount of calories you need to maintain your weight you will have to eat at least 6 meals a day. In effect two breakfasts two lunches and two dinners. What you ate before the surgery for a given meal should be cut in half and eaten at two sittings now. You will more than likely not have an appetite when you leave the hospital, so you will need to eat by the clock., For instances, if you had a sandwich for lunch before the surgery, cut it in half and have half say at 12 noon and the other half at 2:00 PM. You can do the same for breakfast and dinner. Try not to drink fluids with your meal. Your stomach is now reduced in size and filling it with fluids will take the place of the calories you need to maintain your weight and you will not stabilize your weight but continue to lose it if you drink significant amount of fluids with your meals.

The proper way to go forward is to eat a balance diet with enough proteins, carbohydrates and fats to help your body fight against any problems you may encounter.

Please check the chapter on nutrition contained in this guide for further information on this topic.

Sleeping Issues

One of the processes of an esophagectomy is the removal of the sphincter value, which is on top of your stomach. This valve acts like a lid and holds the food in your stomach and without it gravity is the only thing that keeps food from backing up into your esophagus and throat. Because of this, you will need to sleep elevated, at a 30 to 40 degree angle, to avoid aspirating especially during the night when you are asleep.

One way to achieve this required sleeping angle is to buy a medical wedge that will elevate your upper body. You may use an additional pillow on top of the wedge for added height and comfort.

Please check the chapter on sleeping contained in this guide for further information on this topic.

Emotional Issues

The therapies and surgery you have thus far been through is undoubtedly traumatic. If you stay the course, exercise, eat a balanced diet and get the proper sleep you will stand a much greater chance of not experiencing post surgical depression.

In the event that you do find that you may be depressed, it is important for you to see your doctor immediately. Depression may manifest itself in a variety of ways that will usually centers around a lack of motivation. The patient will complain of being tired, not wanting to exercise. They will often ask to be left alone and may tend to sit in front of a television all day. They may not eat properly stating they are not hungry.

Please check the chapter on emotional issues contained in this guide for further information on this topic.

Physical Issues

When you leave the hospital it is quite likely that you will receive a prescription for pain medication to take as needed. Pain medication can have various side effects the most common being constipation. The use of stool softeners and other over the counter medications will help alleviate this issue. The smartest way to offset this is to wean off the pain medication as soon as you can tolerate it. Sometimes an over the counter pain reliever will be sufficient for the pain you are having and that will not have the undesirable side effects. As an added incentive, you will not be able to operate a motor vehicle while taking narcotic pain medication. The sooner you remove the pain medication the sooner you can begin to regain some of the independence you may have lost during therapy. One of the stipulations is as long as you are on pain medication you will not be able to drive a car.

While you were recovering in the hospital, the nurse was likely to be pushing you to exercise, to get up and walk around the floor. In some institutions they let you know how many laps around the floor is a mile and expect you to do that every day you are in the hospital.

That same regimen needs to continue to be part of your daily routine. As outlined in other areas exercise will hasten your overall recovery, help you regain your appetite and keep your mental outlook positive.

Please check the chapter on physical Issues contained in this guide for further information on this topic.

Frequently asked questions

We have captured some frequently asked questions and their responses. We ask that you discuss these responses with your doctor before implementing them.

1. **When I leave the hospital will I go home with a feeding tube and if so how will I take care of it?**
   The decision to place a feeding tube typically is made before surgery, and your surgeon will often discuss with you if he/she intends to place it during your operation and the rationale for doing so. If a feeding tube is placed during or, in some select cases, after surgery, you will most likely go home with it. Tube feedings may or may not be prescribed depending on how well your oral intake is after surgery. A visiting nurse will be arranged to help you and your family learn how to care for the tube and how to manage tube feedings if necessary. Once you have recovered sufficiently and do not need the tube, your surgeon or their staff will remove it in the office.

2. **What kinds of follow up should I have with my surgeon, oncologist or regular physician and has that been set as I leave the hospital?**
   You should see your surgeon soon after being discharged from the hospital. This typically will be in 1-2 weeks after you get home, and you should call the surgeon's office to arrange a time that is mutually convenient. Once you have seen your surgeon

for the immediate postoperative visit, you should also make appointments to follow up with you medical oncologist and family physician in order to keep them informed of your progress. Your surgeon and medical oncologist will coordinate a plan of oncology aftercare and surveillance that will entail periodic visits and scans as necessary.

3. What attitude should I try to have when I leave the hospital?

Having a positive attitude about life in general will help in your recovery process. Take time to stop and smell the roses. Life is precious and we should accept that and live each day to the fullest.

4. Did I receive pain medication when I left the hospital and instructions as to how to use it?

You should have received prescriptions for pain and other medications and instructions from the nurses both about the medication and other aspects of your recovery. Your hospital may or may not allow you to fill your prescriptions prior to leaving so that you have the medication in hand. You should ask your nurse if this is an option so that you do not find yourself without medication because your local pharmacy does not carry the prescribed medicine.

5. How long could I have pain from my Ivor Lewis esophagectomy incision?

After an Ivor Lewis esophagectomy, the patient should expect incision pain to last 4-6 weeks. However, pain medication should help control the pain. You may be able to switch from a prescribed pain medication to an over the counter pain medication. Check with your doctor so as to check the pain you are experiencing and whether or not an over the counter drug will suffice.

6. How long should I stay on the pain medication after I leave the hospital?

As long as you have pain, which can sometimes last approximately 7 to 30 days after surgery. Be aware that prescribed pain medication has a dependency effect if taken over a long period of time. Check with your doctor if you have to renew the prescription for pain medication.

7. How long will the recovery process take?
The recovery process for each patient varies. The average recovery process takes approximately 6-8 weeks.

8. If I am leaving the hospital with stitches, when and where will they be taken out?
Stitches should be removed 10-14 days after surgery in the doctor's office. These are usually staples and they come out without pain to the patient.

9. How important is exercising at this stage of my recovery?
Exercising is one of the most important aspects of this phase of your recovery. A regular routine of walking 1 ½ miles three times a week should be cleared with your doctor.

10. When I get home how will I cope with sleeping on a wedge or adjustable bed or reclining chair?
Getting a good night sleep is important for your recovery process and because they have removed the valve on top of your stomach that acts like a lid to hold your food in your stomach, you will need to sleep on a 30-40 degree angle. You can accomplish this by purchasing a medical wedge from a medical supply store or by buying an adjustable bed. There are other ways to raise the head of your bed to achieve the angle to sleep at. You could put wood boards under the head of the bed so that the entire bed will be elevated. This would put your partner at the same level as you which may not be right for them. You could also buy a reclining chair that will suffice.

11. Did I receive sample menus or nutrition information that will help in my recovery?
The hospital nutritionist will meet with you prior to discharge to review the type of diet and food that you will require following your

operation. They will often have sample menus and/or literature that will help guide you when you go home. If they do not provide any written literature, ask them to provide you some examples as a guide.

12. If there are any other medications that I am going home with do I have the proper instructions on how to use these medications?

You should make sure you completely understand the medications or the prescriptions you are given when you leave the hospital.

13. Will I need to have chemotherapy post surgery?

This will depend on several factors. The biopsy report of the tumor and lymph nodes they took out during the surgery will have an impact on the decision to have post chemotherapy or not. Some oncologists believe that having some post surgical chemotherapy is advisable. You need to discuss this with all of the doctors involved in your case and then you must make the decision as to whether you want to do post surgical treatments.

Chapter 2

NUTRITION

"Learn to enjoy your food as if every meal were a $100 a plate affair"

"Eat to live and not live to eat"

This is the most important chapter in this guide. The need to get enough food into your body to maintain your weight at the beginning of the recovery process and then monitor your food intake to regain some or all of the weight you have loss through the process is your goal. A good proper balanced diet throughout the process will narrow a fair amount of issues you will experience and that should be your goal.

Frequently asked questions

We have captured some frequently asked questions and their responses. We ask that you discuss these responses with your doctor before implementing them.

14. Will I have an appetite when I leave the hospital?

The chances are you will not have an appetite when you leave the hospital. In order to get the proper calories in you to maintain your weight, as this stage of your recovery, you will need to eat by the clock. If it says 12 noon have a half of a sandwich whether you are hungry or not and at 2:00PM have the other half. You will need to do the same for Breakfast and Dinner.

15. Is eating a challenge or will it come easy?

Eating will be a challenge because there are new ways to think about eating then you have done in the past. You need to monitor the amount of food you have at each meal since your stomach is, more than likely, smaller then it was as you remember it and what you will not be able to consume the same amount of food you had in the past and this can become frustrating. Give it time and you will slowly begin to eat more and as the years from surgery extend, you will be able to eat more then you are eating just after surgery.

16. Does my food need to be put through a blender before I eat it?

If you have received the clearance from your doctor to eat solid food you should not put that food through a blender before eating it. You want to exercise your esophagus and chewing food and swallowing it will accomplish this.

17. How will food taste?

The chances are your taste buds have been affected by the process you have just completed. If you had chemo and radiation this will also impact your taste buds and it will be awhile before you will be able to truly taste the food as you did before. Eventually your taste buds will return.

18. Does eating fast affect me?

Definitely. You must eat slowly to get the best out of your food from a nutrition point of view. If you eat fast your stomach will release your food into your digestive track quickly and it can cause you to have diarrhea and other stomach discomfort.

19. Does posture and the clothes I wear impact my digestive system?

You should always sit up straight when you are eating as that allows your food to move into your stomach quicker than if you are slouching and the clothes you wear should be loose fitting around your waist.

20. How many meals a day should I eat?

Because your stomach is smaller as a result of the esophagectomy, you should eat 6 meals a day to get the same number of calories you took in before the surgery, assuming you are not overweight. Some people tend to eat all day with snacks. The key here is to get the number of calories into you that will maintain your current weight and hopefully gain some of the lost weight you have experienced during your ordeal.

21. How much liquid should I take with each meal?

During the meal you should keep your liquid intake down to a minimum. Your stomach is more than likely smaller now so you don't want to be filling it up with liquid and not allowing room for the taking in the calories that the food has. Your full complement of liquids should be taken an hour after your meal.

22. How much liquid should I consume each day?

The normal amount of liquids should be 8-10 glasses of water or green tea or any other liquid that you prefer as your one day goal. Some people find it hard to consume that much liquid during a day and you should do your best to reach this goal.

23. How will milk products affect me?

Patients have been known to experience a lactose-intolerance condition when they go home after surgery. Wait a couple of weeks and try a small amount of milk. If the condition still exists then wait another two weeks and try it again. If you were able to drink milk prior to the surgery you should be able to have it again and it is just a matter of time for your stomach to recognize that.

24. What foods can I eat?

You will be pleased to know that everything that you ate before your surgery can eventually be part of your diet after the surgery. It may take time for your stomach to recognize and hopefully enjoy these foods again. Keep in mind that a balanced diet should be your goal and you should try and achieve this at every meal. By doing this, you will avoid some of the problems you will encounter that are discussed later in this chapter.

25. Should I maintain a food diary?

If patients are experiencing discomfort a day or so after what you have eaten the previous day you may want to keep track of all the food you consume in a day. You can then by trial and error determine what foods are not agreeing with you at the present time and avoid those foods during this part of your recovery. If the foods you determine that are causing you a problem are foods that you were able to tolerate before the surgery, chances are you will be able to eat those again. It is your stomach that is determining this factor and at some point you should be able to eat those foods again.

26. I hear so much about green tea. Should I use it?

Researchers have indicated that the elements in green tea will help you fight cancer and since I want to fight a recurrence if green tea can help me in my fight why not use it. Most of my fluid intake in a given day is green tea. We brew the tea from tea bags as the store bought green tea in bottles has a great deal of sugar which could be harmful. I drink it as ice tea most of the time and there is always a quart of it in the refrigerator when I want it.

27. How much time should I abstain from eating before I go to bed?

You should allow about 2 hours of no food prior to going to bed. You need to allow your stomach ample time to digest your last meal of the day especially if dinner is your largest meal. Acid and bile reflux can occur during your sleep time even if you have elevated your bed to avoid this happening.

28. Are there any foods that I should stay away from before I go to bed?

This question is unique and the answer for each patient could be different. Some patients can't eat chocolate late at night while others can have a bag of potato chips and nothing happens. You need to remember what you ate the previous night if you experience an acid or bile reflux and place that food on your "not to eat late at night" list.

29. Will I ever be able to eat my normal three meals a day and be able to maintain my weight or even gain weight?

As you go further out from your surgery, your stomach will expand somewhat and you will be able to get back to the 3 meals a day with a small snack in between. The quantity of food will increase at a meal but it is important to make sure you eat breakfast, lunch and dinner and not skip a meal as your stomach will not be of a size that you can do this and maintain your weight.

30. Should I take Supplements?

The proper answer to this question is, if you eat a balanced diet you will not need to use supplements unless obviously your doctor says you need to do this to add something your body is not producing or where there is a deficiency. Consulting a doctor who deals with supplements, as his or her field of practice, will assist you in determining if you should take supplements and if so which ones would be right for you. You should not take supplements without first talking to a doctor.

31. Will I be able to go out to dinner and enjoy a meal?

The simple answer to this question is yes. You can go out to dinner post surgery whenever you feel up to it. Recognize that they make doggy bags for a reason and you more than likely would be using them to take home a part of your meal. As you go further out form surgery you will begin to eat more and your taste buds will be back and you will truly enjoy your meal.

32. Can I take glass of wine with dinner?

Again the simple answer is <u>yes, occasionally</u>. Keep in mind that you need to leave a significant amount of room in your stomach to take on the calories of your meal so the more fluid intact you have the less room there is for the food.

33. Did I receive sample menus or nutrition information that will help in my recovery?

The hospital nutritionist will meet with you prior to discharge to review the type of diet and food that you will require following your operation. They will often have sample menus and/or literature that will help guide you when you go home. If they do not provide any written literature, ask them to provide you some examples as a guide.

34. What liquids should I stay away from?

In the immediate <u>postoperative</u> period you should <u>stay away from large amounts of caffeine and alcoh</u>ol, as the former can result in reflux and the latter can interact with your medications. <u>Carbonated beverages can cause abdominal distention and bloating as well</u>. Once you have settled into your dietary routine, and you are farther removed from surgery you can reintroduce the above items slowly.

35. I find my food going down my esophagus slowly. Should this be a concern?

It is very common initially for food to move slowly down your new esophagus for many reasons. First, the new connection between your native esophagus and the new conduit is still a little swollen and thus a little narrow. Second, you will first start with soft foods and transition to bulkier foods, and this takes some getting used to. Be patient, chew your food well and drink plenty of fluids with meals. If after 6 to 8 weeks, food is still going down slowly, or if the swallowing is getting more difficult, notify your surgeon as you may have to have a minor procedure to stretch the new connection.

36. What is dilation?

Sometimes scar tissue develops where the surgeon connected your remaining stomach to your remaining esophagus and this scar tissue can tighten causing the opening to be narrowed and food to go down slowly. If you experience this feeling the first comment is your tumor has not returned. What is needed is for you to contact your surgeon and inform him of this as soon as it begins to happen. He will have you come in and they will do a procedure similar to an endoscopy to stretch the opening and allow you to eat without concern. If you delay and wait too long they will need to do this several times to achieve the proper opening so see your doctor as soon as you have the sensation that food is going down slowly. If you had swallowing problems before the surgery it will seem like that same feeling.

37. I feel bloated after I eat. Is there something I can do to avoid this feeling?

Typically, the sensation of bloating after eating is a result of how much and what is eaten. Remember that you no longer have a stomach with a large reservoir to hold a conventional meal. Chewing your food well, taking plenty of liquids and eating multiple small meals throughout the day will limit feelings of bloating. Also, avoid large amounts of carbonated beverages, such as seltzer or other sodas that can increase the amount of air in the digestive tract.

38. What is dumping syndrome?

Dumping occurs when you eat too many carbohydrates and/ or fats and not a balanced meal. This condition can develop a short time after you eat or it can happen several hours after you eat. Your stomach, in effect, is saying I can't handle the amount of carbohydrates and/or fats you are taking in and it opens the lower valve in your stomach and flushes all of the food into your intestines. At that time your pancreas is shooting insulin into your blood stream to help with the digestive process and there is no food in your stomach so it causes you to have what they call a low sugar reaction. You will feel an overall weakness, sweaty and heart palpitations. You may experience diarrhea as a result of this episode.

It is a reminder that you should eat a balanced meal using all food groups to avoid this dumping syndrome.

39. What do I do when a dumping episode occurs?

If you take some orange juice or something sweet and eat some protein like nuts the feeling should go away in about 20-30 minutes. If it does not please consult your doctor.

Chapter 3

SLEEPING

"You are unique and sometimes you need to improvise for best results."

Next to the nutrition chapter this chapter gains the most importance as not securing a proper amount of sleep will impact all that you do. It is important that you get a good night sleep and however you accomplish that is the right way for you. Everyone is unique and what works for someone may not work for another. You are in control and if sleeping on a wedge, or an adjustable bed or a reclining chair works for you that is what you should do.

Frequently asked questions

We have captured some frequently asked questions and their responses. We ask that you discuss these responses with your doctor before implementing them.

40. Why do I need to sleep on an angle?

When they performed the esophagectomy they would have, in most cases, removed the valve on top of your stomach so in effect you do not have a lid on your stomach to keep the contents in your stomach in your stomach. You need to sleep on this 30 to 40 degree angle to achieve this goal. If you don't then what is in your stomach will roll up into your throat and you could aspirate which can be a major problem.

41. What are the ways that I can achieve this 30 to 40 degree angle while I sleep?

There are several conventional ways to achieve this angle and there are some home remedies as well:

◆ **MEDICAL WEDGES**

They sell medical wedges that will be the proper angle and if you place a pillow on top of the wedge you will be able to sleep without complications. During the night you may find yourself slipping down the wedge and when this happens you could have a reflux experience. Some people have put pillows under their knees to prevent the sliding, if this continues you should find an alternative method indicated in this chapter.

◆ **ADJUSTABLE BEDS**

This alternative usually works because you can raise the top of the bed a sufficient amount to achieve the desired degree angle and you can raise the foot portion of the adjustable bed high enough so you won't slip during the night. You can buy an adjustable bed for yourself and your partner and your partner can keep their bed at one angle and yours at another. When you are not sleeping the beds can be made to look like one king size bed and give your bedroom that appearance.

◆ **RECLINING CHAIR**

Some people have indicated that they get the best night sleep using a reclining chair. The arms of the chair act as a restraint from turning in your sleep and therefore the possibility of getting into a position that would cause acid or bile reflux would be remote. Having one in your bedroom gives you the flexibility of choosing where you sleep without leaving your bedroom.

42. Where can I get an adjustable bed?

Most good bedding stores will have adjustable beds for sale. You need to find one that is comfortable for you. The best approach is to look on your internet and determine the stores near you and shop prices.

43. Does my health insurance cover my adjustable bed costs?

There are insurance companies that have agreed, we are told, to cover the cost or a part thereof of an adjustable bed for esophageal cancer patients. You need to contact your insurance company and present the question to them.

44. What do I do when I travel? How will I achieve this desired 30-40 degree level?

They do make an inflatable wedge and it usually will come in its own pouch and have a small pump with it as well. This fits well into your suitcase and when you arrive at the hotel you can inflate the wedge and use it in any bed. You can easily deflate it and return it to your suitcase for your trip home.

45. Where can I get an inflatable wedge?

Most medical supply companies will carry an inflatable wedge. You should look at the internet and determine those stores near you that carry adjustable wedges and then shop for the one that you find fits your needs and you can manage.

46. Does my health insurance cover my inflatable wedge cost?

There are insurance companies that have agreed, we are told, to cover the cost or a part thereof of an inflatable wedge for esophageal cancer patients. You need to contact your insurance company and present the question to them.

47. Can I sleep on my side?

Everyone has a different healing process after esophagectomy. Some people will be able to sleep on their side and some people will not. If you develop coughing while laying on one side or the other, you may be experiencing aspiration (inhalation of gastrointestinal contents into your airway) and have to stop sleeping on that particular side. Some people may develop acid or bile reflux and have difficulty sleeping any way other than with their head and back elevated on pillows or wedges. Others may have had a large incision in their right chest (called a thoracotomy) and not be able to sleep on that side until they have healed and their pain at the incision sight has decreased.

48. Can I sleep on my stomach?

This is extremely difficult to do because of the pressure it puts on your chest and stomach which can make it difficult to sleep. If you have slept on your stomach in the past you should try it and see how comfortable you are. All of your sleeping focus should be in getting a good night sleep and whatever you can do to achieve that is acceptable.

49. I am tired after I eat a meal. Should I lay-down and rest?

Eating a big meal will cause you to feel tired and you want to lay-down and rest. Most people can do this. However be aware of reflux and it could occur after you have eaten while you are at rest. Maintain the 30-40 degree angle while you rest.

Chapter 4

EMOTIONAL ISSUES

"Having a positive attitude about life in general will help in your recovery process. Take time to stop and smell the roses.

Life is precious and we should accept that and live each day to the fullest"

When we think about the emotional side of this disease we find people may tend to overlook the signs that your emotional side is playing a major role either negatively or positively in your recovery process. In this chapter we try to highlight those areas that are a concern and what you can do to address them.

At this point in your recovery, depression is a very real threat. You and your caretaker need to be on watch for signs that depression is setting in. Exercising is a way to overcome early levels of depression. If it persists you should see your doctor immediately.

Frequently asked questions

We have captured some frequently asked questions and their responses. We ask that you discuss these responses with your doctor before implementing them.

50. Can I become depressed when I return home from the hospital?

You have just experienced a life-changing diagnosis and treatment, and both your body and mind are adjusting to new realities. Living with cancer brings you face to face with mortality. Changes in your family and occupational roles may occur. For some, money and legal concerns may increase. With changes in your body, with altered life roles, and with concern about what the future holds, a cancer diagnosis is disorienting. Feelings of sadness, confusion and fear naturally arise. Difficulties eating and sleeping after the surgery may add to feelings of unease and distress. If feelings of sadness or irritability persist over many days, or if the feelings interfere with ability to your function at work or home, you may be experiencing an episode of depression. The American Cancer Society reports that about 25% of cancer patients at some point experience depression. Both men and women diagnosed with cancer can become depressed at equal rates.

51. What are symptoms of depression?

A loss of motivation and energy are central to an episode of depression. Feelings may include sadness and emptiness, or increased irritability.

Previously enjoyed activities, work or relationships may hold little or no interest. Friends and family members may notice these changes, and find it more difficult to engage their loved one who is depressed. If depression becomes more severe, a sense of hopelessness may spiral into suicidal thoughts. Problems in clear, rational thinking in a state of depression can also occur. Additionally, changes in eating or sleeping are common during an episode of depression.

Identifying the emergence of depression can be challenging following surgery. Problematically, the symptoms of depression significantly overlap the physical challenges following surgical recovery including low energy, difficulties with sleep and diminished appetite. These overlapping symptoms of surgical recovery and depression can lead to under-diagnosis and treatment of the mood disorder. Further complicating matters is the stigma associated with psychiatric disorders. An individual may perceive his or her depression as an indication of weakness, rather than as a treatable brain disorder.

Depression in cancer patients occurs to a greater extent for those who have experienced a previous episode of depression or anxiety. Depression is also more common in individuals with a more advanced stage of cancer, and those who experience medical complications during recovery. Because depression is so prevalent, screening for a mood disorder should be a part of your follow-up visits with your medical team. If at any time, you or your family members are concerned about depression; your doctor should be consulted.

52. What Treatments are available for depression?

Research shows that psychological treatment, medication and exercise can help you overcome depression. Anti-depressant medication can be helpful in treating symptoms of both depression and anxiety. Individual and/or family therapy can be helpful in providing support, dealing with the many changes in your body and life at this time, and improving your mood. For mild depression, regular exercise has been shown to be as effective as medication in reducing symptoms. Walking three times a week for a half hour each time has been shown to be helpful in reducing symptoms. Daily walks for a half hour are even better.

Regular sleeping and good nutrition are also helpful in recovering from depression. Of course, post-surgery, the changes in your body can make a stable pattern of eating, exercising, and sleeping challenging.

Joining a support group can be especially important in normalizing the many challenges you are experiencing. In a support group you can learn from others, reflect, and share your own experiences. Group membership can help provide meaning and validation at a time of great change in your life.

53. How can I stay positive during my recovery?

This is a time in life when you need positive relationships and experiences. You may, perhaps for one of the first times in life, give yourself permission to move towards what makes you happiest. Staying close to family and friends who can offer support is important. You may find yourself wanting to offer support to others to add to your sense of meaning and purpose.

As you feel stronger, returning to activities that you have enjoyed throughout your life can feel grounding. While many things have irrecoverably changed in your life, staying connected to work or recreational activities that you have enjoyed over many years can add a sense of comfort. Taking care of yourself, and making that a priority, is essential. New ways of eating and sleeping as you recover from surgery can be thought of as a way to nurture your body post-surgery.

From an emotional perspective, you can expect to not always feel positive Pain, suffering and worry are a part of life, and you may feel these and other negative emotions at times more than you ever have before. Expecting yourself to be perfect, or perfectly positive, is unrealistic, and will ultimately add to your sense of suffering. That being said, this is not a time in life for toughing it out alone. It's important to find people to talk to about your difficult times and feelings. Having supportive relationships to help you deal with these negative thoughts will go a long way. Panic attacks can be another manifestation of anxiety. A panic attack starts suddenly with symptoms of a racing heart, shortness of breath, and tingling. The feeling of anxiety is strong, and during a panic attack there is a felt need to escape. Temperature sensations of chills or hot flashes may accompany the anxiety. Episodes of panic disorders are discrete, but between episodes there is often dread of another occurrence. An individual with panic disorder may begin to change their behaviors in an attempt to avoid another attack. For example, someone might avoid leaving the house, or driving for fear of having another attack. For some, anxiety predates the cancer diagnosis and for others anxiety occurs for the first time following cancer. Either way, anxiety is treatable by cognitive-behavioral therapy, often in conjunction with medication. In therapy, an individual re-learns to relax her or his mind and body in response to anxiety-arousing thoughts or situations. Therapy also offers support to deal with the medical and emotional issues that may underlie anxiety. Meditation and breathing techniques can also be very helpful in reducing anxiety.

55. I am having problems with sexual interest and activity. What should I do?

Physical and emotional factors can affect sexual interest for patients recovering from surgery. Following surgical treatment, your body is changed. Basic life functions of breathing, especially during physical exertion, eating and sleeping are impacted. Body image may be affected by surgery. There may be anxiety on the part of both partners of doing physical harm during sexual activity. Both partners may need assurance from the doctor regarding sexual activity post-surgery.

Emotionally, there can be many distractions that interfere with sexual interest. Financial worries, concerns about one's health and the future, occupational concerns and more can preoccupy thinking and crowd out sexual interest. Anxiety may take a toll on sexual motivation for both partners.

Physical closeness and intimacy can be an important part of healing for both you and your partner. Taking things slowly and gaining comfort with gentle forms of touching can bring you closer. Communicating your concerns to each other is an important form of connection that can lead to exploration and growth in your relationship.

56. I continue to think about a recurrence. Is that normal? How do I handle the possibility of recurrence?

Of the many concerns that you have at this juncture, surely the worry of recurrence is one of the most difficult. Facing the possibility of recurrence brings one close to the prospect of physical suffering and death. While we turn away from the reality of death in our culture, when one is facing the possibility of cancer recurrence this strategy of avoidance is no longer effective or even possible. Thinking about a recurrence is natural, and in fact is the mind's way of preparing for all possibilities.

Having a spiritual view of one's meaning and purpose in life can be helpful when facing an uncertain future. You may choose to spend time reflecting on what is most important to you. Finding others who are also experiencing uncertainty following a diagnosis of cancer can bring comfort, and reduce a sense of fear and isolation. Sharing your feelings, and fears, with loved ones provides further opportunities for support. It is also important to discuss your fears with your doctors and seek professional help. Having an understanding of the success of your therapy and professional guidance can be helpful in reducing your level of stress in this area.

Should a recurrence occur please check the Chapter on Physical Issues to see questions and answers dealing with this topic.

57. I feel a lack of interest in taking charge of my journey through the recovery process. Should I be concerned?

It is very important that you bring a very positive person to your recovery process. Each day is a new experience and you need to have a goal for that day and look to achieve it. If it is exercising then you should find the time to exercise that day. Setting goals and achieving them will be an added plus in your recovery process.

58. Will I ever feel normal again?

This is an interesting question as it relies on your definition of normal. The process you have gone through and the adjustments you have had to make in eating and sleeping have to be considered the New Normal but when you think about it eating smaller meals is recommended by nutritionists as what all people should follow and sleeping on an incline is also recommended for everyone so you see the "New Normal" Is what most people wanting a better health should follow.

59. How should I approach life once I am home from the hospital?

We live in a world that seems to be consumed with worry. We live in a world that focuses on "what ifs". Life is precious and there is no better way to understand that principal then to see nature in all its glory. Watching a sunrise or sun set will be a positive experience and take the time to look at the world outside your door. Someone once said," Stop and smell the roses". Live life each day to the fullest and try and "Make where you are better because you are there".

60. What role does my spiritual side play in my recovery process?

We may think this is a difficult question to answer given our confidence with where our spiritual life is at, at this time. If we have not had a spiritual life, we may think turning to that now may be difficult to do.

Regardless of the God you pray to we know he is a loving and caring God and welcomes you with open and gentle hands.

A saying that has been used is, "God sits on my right shoulder and there is nothing that He and I together can't handle".

61. What role should my family play in my recovery process?

It is important that you allow your family to express their love for you in this time. The relationship environment that the family generates can be a major influence in the healing process and involving the family is important to them and to you. Watching your children and grandchildren grow and approach the world's challenges will help you realize the importance of life and it will help you take on your challenges and succeed.

62. Does my positive or negative thinking impact my recovery?

It is extremely important that you remain positive throughout your recovery process and for life in general. Doctors will tell you that a positive person will have a better outcome then one that does not share this approach. Doctors will tell you that a person is made up of three parts namely, His Mind, Body and Spirit, and although they are responsible for making the body better they have a major influence in making sure the Mind and Spirit of the person in their care is equally addressed.

63. What is the course of action once a recurrence is determined?

Once recurrence is suspected or established, evaluation of the extent of recurrence and need for additional confirmation with biopsies is needed. Locally recurrent disease only can sometimes be treated with surgery or radiation based therapy. More commonly recurrence after primary local therapy involves distant metastatic disease, which cannot generally be treated by potentially curative surgery or radiotherapy. Systemic chemotherapy is usually the appropriate next step in care.

64. How many difference chemo drugs are available to the Oncologist in determining the plan for a specific patient?

There are 5-6 classes of common chemotherapy agents used to treat recurrent esophageal cancer, including 5-FU drugs, platinum agents, taxanes, irinotecan, mitomycin, and anthracyclines. The choice of a single agent versus combination chemotherapy program is dependent on the ability of the individual patient to tolerate therapy, as well as the severity of the recurrence and degree of symptoms or debility that the patient experiences. A new drug herceptin may be appropriate to use in combination with chemotherapy in patients whose tumor tests positive for HER2 expression.

65. Are there research projects that are close that will be a breakthrough with esophageal cancer recurrences?

Ongoing clinical trials are evaluating new agents in the context of phase I, II and III trials. The availability of and advisability of entrance into any such trials needs to be reviewed with each individual patient.

66. Have certain drugs shown promise in this area?

Other than herceptin, no new agents are near approval for esophageal cancer.

67. Are there other countries outside of the United States that are addressing prevention of recurrence projects?

Trials are ongoing globally to treat esophageal cancer, but it is unlikely that travel abroad will be advisable to pursue such therapy as there are no new treatments that appear promising enough to undertake overseas travel.

68. I find it hard to concentrate. How do I correct this?

There are many reasons why you may have a hard time concentrating in the post-operative period. Esophagectomy is a major surgery causing significant stress on your body. Your body will need time to recover from this stress. A variety of factors such as your pain medication and oral intake of fluids and food may be affecting your concentration levels. All patients are discharged from the hospital with pain medication. These pain medications often include opiates such as oxycodone. Opiates may affect your concentration level and can make you feel sleepy. It is possible that you may need to have your pain medication regimen changed if your concentration difficulties are especially disturbing to you.

Another factor relating to concentration is the level of sugar (glucose) in your blood. Our brain requires large amounts of energy for its many jobs. Because you have had a surgery that changes your gastrointestinal tract, your eating patterns may change. You may require more frequent but smaller meals. It is very important that you continue to eat and drink regardless of whether you have lost your appetite or not. Scheduling small meals and snacks throughout the day may help your concentration because you are providing your brain with a more steady supply of energy. If you are diabetic, you may need to have your diabetes medications changed because your eating patterns have changed. If you have diabetes and experience problems with your concentration, let your primary care provider and surgical team know about this.

69. I can't seem to read and retain what I am reading. Is this normal?

It is normal to have slight difficulties with mental tasks such as reading and short-term memory in the post-operative period. These difficulties are likely related to your pain medications as well as your overall healing process. It is possible that you may need to have changes made to your pain medication regimen as opiate pain medications can affect your mental sharpness. However, you should give yourself a few weeks after surgery to feel closer to your pre-surgery self. You may require more sleep, food, and rest to heal from surgery.

Chapter 5

PHYSICAL ISSUES

"Life is precious and we should accept that and live each day to the fullest"

In this chapter we will focus on issues that you may encounter from a physical point of view. Obviously the chapters dealing with nutrition and exercising play a major role in getting your body strong and back to the way it was prior to your surgery.

The key to a good recovery is keeping your Body along with your Mind and Spirit headed in a positive direction. A good physical presence will give you a good feeling about yourself and will make the recovery process move quickly along.

Frequently asked questions

We have captured some frequently asked questions and their responses. We ask that you discuss these responses with your doctor before implementing them.

70. **What will happen if I pick up something heavy?**
It is strongly advised that a patient not lift anything heavy while recovering from surgery for three months. A hernia may develop in the incision if you do so.

71. **I have nausea. Is there a medicine I can take?**
Patients can take a prescription medication for nausea. Reglan or Zofran are very commonly prescribed.

72. **I have a shortness of breath when I bend over? Is there something I can do to eliminate this shortness of breath?**
Since they have pulled your stomach up to attach to your remaining esophagus they have created less room in your chest cavity for your heart and lungs. If you overeat you may feel this shortness of breath because your lungs are fighting for space that is now occupied by your stomach and this may cause a shortness of breath. Exercise after you eat may be difficult because you are full but eventually exercise will help you with this condition.

73. What is neuropathy?

Neuropathy is nerve injury, which happens after chest incisions. Symptoms of neuropathy may include pain, numbness and decrease sensation, tingling and burning. If you experience this condition speak to your doctor and decide on a course of action to be taken.

74. Will I have to take antacids after surgery?

The surgery should have removed one of the acid producing glands and the amount of acid or bile that you produce post esophagectomy should be less then you did before the surgery. If acid or bile reflux occurs after your esophagectomy make sure you are leaving ample time between your last meal and going to bed each night. If you feel that you are doing this then ask your doctor as to which antacid you should take. You may be able to use an over the counter drug or if your doctor thinks a prescribed medicine would be better for you than that is the way to go.

75. I am constipated. What do I do?

If the patient is constipated, we recommend that they take a laxative and/or stool softener and try to decrease narcotic use. Usually this occurs when you are on pain medication as this is one of the side effects of that drug.

76. I have the sweats. What do I do?

Sweats can be the product of a dumping syndrome which is explained in another section of this guide. Take your temperature. If it is above normal, call your doctor and speak to him/her about this condition and what may have precipitated the sweats.

77. I have vomiting after meals. What do I do to correct this?

You should eat small, soft meals and decrease the quantity of food. If it persists, call your doctor because you may have a stricture that may be easily corrected by dilation. Please see the question on dilation to understand what this procedure is and what it accomplishes.

78. I have swelling of my hands and feet. What should I do?

Swelling of the hands and feet are normal after an esophagectomy. There is nothing that needs to be done, it will go away in time. We do recommend that you walk as much as possible and raise your legs above your heart when lying down. If this condition persists call your doctor, as there may be other things happening that would warrant your doctor's attention.

79. I have dizziness. What should I do?

If you feel dizzy during recovery, drink plenty of fluids and take the time to sit and rest. Make sure you are eating a balanced diet and eating all the meals you should be eating. If it persists please call your doctor and inform him what you are experiencing.

80. I have mouth sores. What should I do?

It is recommended to mix salt or peroxide with water rinse your mouth out with water. Sometimes thrush, a fungal infection, may result which requires a special mouthwash. If persistent, show your doctor.

81. I have restless leg syndrome. What should I do?

Exercise regularly, decrease caffeine, alcohol and tobacco use, do leg stretching, walk, and apply heat or cold to the legs. Also, a pillow should be put between the knees when lying down.

82. I am running a temperature of 99.6. What should I do?

Your body fluctuates through a range of temperatures throughout the day as it adapts to its environment. A temperature of at least 101.5°F is required for it to be considered a true fever. However, in the post-esophagectomy situation, it would be best to let your surgeon and his or her team know if you have a temperature at or above 100°F as it may indicate that you are developing a leak where your "new esophagus" (known as the anastomosis) was created in your chest or neck. You should also note whether any of your incisions have become red, hot, tender, or draining as it could also be an early warning sign of surgical site infection.

83. What do I do if I feel tightness in my chest?

Chest tightness is a symptom that should always be reported to your surgeon and his or her team. The sensation of tightness in your chest in the post-operative period may signal something concerning, such as a myocardial infarction (also known as a heart attack). However, it may also be an indication of something more benign in nature such as the normal healing process of your wounds. If chest tightness is associated with swallowing, it could indicate the development of a stricture (an area of tightness) at the anastomosis (connection) of your "new esophagus." If you have chest tightness associated with pain or crushing pressure in the chest that may move toward the jaw or arm, you should go immediately to your local emergency department or call 911. Other symptoms such as difficulty breathing, nausea, dizziness and lightheadedness in conjunction with significant chest tightness are another indication that you should go to your local emergency department or call 911.

84. If I get the chills with or without a fever, what should I do?

Chills are when your body shakes or shivers, and are an involuntary contraction of muscles in response to fluctuations in body temperature. If you develop chills you should take your temperature. You should then call your surgeon or his/her team of healthcare providers and speak with them about this. Although chills may be benign in nature, they also could be an indication that you have developed an infection in your body, such as a surgical site infection, urinary tract infection, pneumonia, or infection in your blood (sepsis).

85. How long until I can travel by plane after my surgery?

After esophagectomy, there is concern that in the immediate post-operative period air travel could make you more prone to conditions called pneumothorax and pneumomediastinum. Pneumothorax and pneumomediastinum are conditions in which air is trapped outside of the lung or around the heart. Both of these may be dangerous conditions. Air travel causes increased pressure inside the lungs, which may damage the healing tissues in your lungs and around your heart. It is unknown how long a patient should wait before air travel after an esophagectomy and each surgeon will have their own opinion on this question. Your surgeon will probably ask you to wait anywhere from 2 to six weeks to safely fly after your esophagectomy.

86. I have a cough after meals. Why is this and what can I do to correct it?

Coughing after meals is an indication you may be aspirating (inhaling) contents from your gastrointestinal tract into your lungs. Surgery on the esophagus is a predisposing factor to aspiration. This is just like when you have food or water "go down the wrong pipe" causing you to cough. Be sure to sit straight up in a chair when eating all meals. You should talk to your surgeon and his or her team about this problem if you are experiencing coughing after meals. They may make recommendations such as eating with your chin down towards your chest; avoiding certain types of foods such as thin liquids; or even refer you to a speech pathologist to work with you on your swallowing.

87. When I touch my incisions I feel a tingling feeling. Is this normal?

It is common to have numbness, tingling or pain at or near your incisions as a result of nerve irritation. This usually resolves substantially if not completely over several weeks following the operation.

88. Will I have a cough and if so what should I do?

A dry cough can develop as part of the post surgical recovery and will usually resolve over time. If the cough is productive of colored sputum and/or is associated with a temperature above 101.5°F, you should inform your surgeon's office.

89. What is an incision hernia?

An incision hernia is an area of weakness of the inner strength layer of the abdominal wall because of inadequate healing. This results in bulging especially when you bear down or cough. It may require repair depending on the size and what symptoms are associated with it. If you think you may have a hernia, call or bring it to your surgeon's attention during one of your follow up visits.

90. What is hydration and how important is it to my recovery process?

Hydration is the process of taking in fluids, and it is important for many reasons. First, adequate hydration is necessary to maintain good blood pressure and blood flow to all of your vital organs. Second, taking in enough liquids helps swallowing and digestion. Third, maintaining good fluid intake helps you avoid constipation, particularly in your recovery from surgery when you may be taking narcotics. Good sources of hydration include water, juice, and electrolyte solutions such as Gatorade or any similar drink. Avoid caffeinated products as your sole source of fluid intake.

91. I have dry mouth. What do I do?

Dry mouth can results from a number of causes. The most common is from dehydration, so make sure that you are ingesting plenty of liquids. If you are using oxygen at home, make sure it is humidified as it can dry out your nasal and oral passages. Certain medications are associated with dry mouth, so check with your doctor.

92. I have problem with urination. What should I do?

There are many types of urination problems, including inability to start, incontinence, frequent urination, burning on urination and inability to empty your bladder completely. You should call your doctor and describe the difficulty. Once again, infrequent and concentrated urine may be the result of dehydration, so adequate fluid intake is critical.

Frequency, burning and foul-smelling urination may be indicative of a urinary infection.

93. I have numbness and tingling of my hands and feet. What should I do?

Numbness and tingling of the extremities can result from a number of causes. If you have had pre-surgical chemotherapy and the numbness and tingling is on both sides of your body and predates your operation, it may be a side effect of your chemotherapy drugs, and you should contact your medical oncologist. If the symptoms are on one side, then it may be related to your position during your operation, and you should talk with your surgeon's office. If the numbness and tingling is associated with coldness of the limb and skin discoloration, contact your doctor immediately.

94. I continue to have reflux when I sleep. What should I do?

Reflux after esophageal cancer surgery is common because the normal sphincters (muscle barriers to reflux) have been disabled, and gravity plays a larger role in emptying of the upper digestive tract. There are many things you can do to limit reflux during sleep. First, avoid eating or meals close to bedtime. Second, avoid laying flat while sleeping and make sure the head of your bed is elevated at 30°. This is best achieved by placing a wedge underneath the head of your bed—this can be purchased at any health supply store.

95. When I go home, how long before I am able to drive a car?

Complete healing typically takes 4-6 weeks following surgery. A good rule of thumb regarding driving a car or doing any activity that requires periods of concentration and good reflex time is to engage in it once you are taking no more narcotic pain pills in a day. Above all, use common sense and do not attempt to drive if you are still having significant pain or fatigue throughout the day.

Chapter 6

CONCLUSION

"Make where you are better because you are there"

This guide is a work in progress. We hope you have been helped with the issues raised and discussed in this guide as you journey through the recovery process. Its goal was to be of assistance to you and reduce hopefully some of the anxiety and concern you may have as you encounter an issue in your recovery process.

If you should experience an issue that is not reflected in this guide we ask that you inform us of that issue and what you have done to confront and overcome that issue. Please send an email to us at info@fightec.org or write to us at ECEF, PO BOX 821, Manalapan NJ 07726.

Frequently asked questions

We have captured some frequently asked questions and their responses. We ask that you discuss these responses with your doctor before implementing them.

96. How can I be of help in getting the message out to the public that this disease exists?

ECEF has a program called a Family Awareness Program in which you, with the help of ECEF, can write a letter to all of your family, friends and business associates telling them about this disease and telling them what symptoms they should be aware of such as heartburn, smoking or heavy drinking.

97. Where can I find assistance as I journey through this process?

The first call you should make should be to your physician and ask him about your question. If it is a quality of life question you can contact, The Esophageal Cancer Education Foundation (ECEF) provides a group of services that you can take advantage of that will assist you through your recovery process. Go to our web site www.fightec.org and click on the SERVICE button and you will see what we offer, all at no cost to you.

98. How do I live the rest of my life?

Simply stated, one day at a time. Each day can be a positive experience and you need to focus on that aspect and live each day to the fullest.

99. What sayings can I look at to determine if there is one that fits my needs?

We have indicated throughout this guide various sayings and catch phrases that you can lock into and recall as your journey continues each day. Sometimes when you think of an unanswerable question you may recall one of these sayings and say it in response each time that question comes up. People will ask do you think about recurrences and we tell them almost every day and when they ask me what do I say or how do I respond I say "God sits on my right shoulder and there is nothing that He and I together can't handle"

Hopefully one of these may be of help in a difficult time:
- *Stop and Smell the Roses*
- *Make where you are better because you are there.*
- *My life is a gift from God and what I do with that life is my gift to Him.*
- *Life is precious, enjoy each moment.*
- *Eat to live and not live to eat*

100. What do you think of this guide?

We ask that you help us make this guide better for the patients and caregivers that will see it in the future. If there are any issues that you have encountered that are not shown in this guide please write to us at info@figtec.org and share the issue and what you have done to overcome that issue. If there are issues in this guide that you have experienced with a result that you would like to share with us please do by writing to us at info@fightec.org. We certainly welcome your opinion of this guide and wish you nothing but positive experiences as your journey continues through the recovery process.